Baby Blues

A Naturopathic Approach
for Postpartum Health

Dr. Nancy Lins, ND

BALBOA
PRESS
A DIVISION OF HAY HOUSE

For Chiyana

all my Love

Balboa Press books may be ordered through booksellers or by contacting:

Balboa Press
A Division of Hay House
1663 Liberty Drive
Bloomington, IN 47403
www.balboapress.com
1 (877) 407-4847

Because of the dynamic nature of the Internet, any web addresses or
links contained in this book may have changed since publication and
may no longer be valid. The views expressed in this work are solely those
of the author and do not necessarily reflect the views of the publisher,
and the publisher hereby disclaims any responsibility for them.

The author of this book does not dispense medical advice or prescribe the use
of any technique as a form of treatment for physical, emotional, or medical
problems without the advice of a physician, either directly or indirectly. The
intent of the author is only to offer information of a general nature to help
you in your quest for emotional and spiritual well-being. In the event you use
any of the information in this book for yourself, which is your constitutional
right, the author and the publisher assume no responsibility for your actions.

Any people depicted in stock imagery provided by Thinkstock are models,
and such images are being used for illustrative purposes only.
Certain stock imagery © Thinkstock.

Print information available on the last page.

ISBN: 978-1-5043-4388-6 (sc)
ISBN: 978-1-5043-4390-9 (hc)
ISBN: 978-1-5043-4389-3 (e)

Library of Congress Control Number: 2015918705

Balboa Press rev. date: 12/31/2015

This book is dedicated to all the women who suffer with postpartum mood disorders, their families, and their doctors.

Contents

Acknowledgments

I would like to thank my teachers of naturopathic medicine who gave me the strong foundation for the work in this book.

I especially thank:

Dr. Katherine Leonardi for her constant support and encouragement;

Dr. Anne-Marie Lambert for her clinical expertise and kind heart;

my husband, Lee Lins, for being my solid rock and biggest promoter;

my children, Dalton and Ciana, for being my greatest teachers;

and universal intelligence, from which all things flow.

Introduction

*A healthy person is a happy person and a happy person
is a healthy person.*

—Deepak Chopra

Postpartum depression (PPD) is a serious medical condition estimated to affect one in eight women who give birth. It can also affect women who have a miscarriage or other loss of pregnancy. The causes of PPD can be both physical and emotional.

Physically, the drop in progesterone levels in the body after the placenta is delivered can cause depression for women who are hormonally sensitive. Breast-feeding may be difficult for some women, leading to feelings of inadequacy as a mother. The hormone prolactin, which causes lactation, is also thought to contribute to depression in some women.

An idealized expectation of having a perfect, natural birth experience—that instead turns out to be a highly medicalized birth ending in a C-section—can be both physically and emotionally devastating for a woman. The weeks of recovery from surgery and other complications may lead to depression or anxiety disorders. A new mother may mourn the loss of her dream birth experience and feel angry or disappointed.

Women treated for infertility may also have a higher risk of PPD for hormonal reasons. They often have had extensive medical intervention with the use of strong hormonal treatments in order to become pregnant. There may be fear in trusting the body's wisdom. The underlying causes of infertility may have never been addressed, leading to an increased risk of PPD.

Emotionally, some women just don't feel normal after giving birth. A history of emotional or mental disorders will add to their risk. Stressful life events, negative birth experiences, and poor practical or emotional support from family or friends can also increase their chances of suffering from PPD.

"Baby Blues" vs. PPD

Most women (70–80 percent) will experience "baby blues" beginning a few days or weeks postpartum. Symptoms can include irritability, mood swings, crying spells, feelings of tension or nervousness, sleep disturbance, feelings of being overwhelmed, loss of appetite, and sadness. Baby blues generally lasts anywhere from a few hours to a few days and is caused by the sudden fluctuation of hormones following the birth. The condition usually goes away quickly without treatment.

On the other hand, postpartum mood disorder (PPMD) can include the above symptoms, but it doesn't resolve quickly. Symptoms can develop anytime during the first year, but they generally occur during the first three to six months following the birth. Other symptoms include the following: strong feelings of dejection, anger, guilt, anxiety, exhaustion, memory loss, depression, paranoia, inability to concentrate, feelings of hopelessness and inadequacy, inability to cope, guilt, despair, loss of concern or overconcern for the baby, panic attacks, fears of going insane, strange and violent thoughts, thoughts of death or suicide, fears of hurting the baby, loss of interest in pleasurable activities, loss of sex drive, loss of cognitive function, and insomnia. These symptoms can take up to one year to develop.

Early warning signs of PPD include difficulty bonding with the baby, thoughts of giving the baby away or wishing it didn't exist, not wanting to hold or care for the baby, or not being able to care for oneself. The possibility of recurrence with future pregnancies is estimated to be 60-80 percent.

On the far side of the spectrum of postpartum disorders is *postpartum psychosis*. Psychosis occurs in less than 2 percent of women, and symptoms may include delusional thoughts, hallucinations, and hearing voices. This serious condition requires immediate medical attention. The mother and her children may be at risk for injury. Psychosis has a 25 percent chance of recurring with future pregnancies.

Naturopathic Medicine

This book describes naturopathic principles. The paradigm of naturopathic medicine is based on uncovering and removing the *cause* of disease, while the conventional medical approach usually focuses on removing the *symptoms*. In the long run, a condition may become chronic and cause serious harm to the body. Naturopathic medicine is not a Band-Aid approach to health, but rather a holistic model for health and healing based on the following naturopathic physician's oath:

Naturopathic Physician's Oath

Primum Non Nocere
First of all, to do no harm

Vis Medicatrix Naturae
To act in cooperation with the healing power of nature

Tolle Causam
To address the fundamental causes of disease

Tolle Totum
To heal the whole person through individualized treatment

Docere
To teach principles of healthy living and preventative medicine

Chapter 1

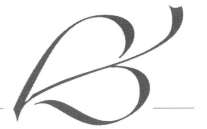

Achieving Hormonal Balance

What we feel and think and are, is to a great extent determined by the state of our ductless glands and viscera.

—Aldous Huxley

The sudden drop in progesterone levels following birth is a major cause of PPMD. Not all women are hormonally sensitive, but for those who are, this biochemical shift can be quite dramatic. Women who have experienced PMS symptoms with their menstrual cycles are more susceptible to PPMD.

During pregnancy, the placenta produces high levels of progesterone to sustain the pregnancy. Once the placenta (the afterbirth) is delivered, the progesterone levels plummet. For this reason, it's important to look at progesterone levels first. A physician who specializes in complementary and alternative medicine (CAM) is your best choice. He or she may be a naturopathic doctor (ND), medical doctor (MD), or osteopathic doctor (DO) trained in natural or bioidentical hormone therapies.

Progesterone Deficiency

Signs and symptoms of a progesterone deficiency may include amenorrhea (not resuming a period), anxiety, hot flashes, night sweats, insomnia, confusion, depression, and dizzy spells. If the period has returned, the signs will be similar to premenstrual syndrome (PMS) and may include irritability, abdominal bloating and cramping, headaches before the period, moodiness, hopelessness, food cravings, sadness and crying easily. Some women will not have PMS before the pregnancy but will develop it after giving birth. Severe PMS is called PMDD or *premenstrual dysphoric disorder* and is sometimes treated with antidepressant medications.

Progesterone Testing

Progesterone testing may initially be conducted using saliva or blood samples. If the woman is not cycling and menses has not returned, only one sample is necessary. If she is cycling, a single blood or saliva sample may be taken on the twenty-first day. The chart below shows a series of multiple saliva samples taken for an entire month. This report gives the most complete information about the cycling of women's hormone levels.

Sample of Female Hormone Panel

eFHP	Expanded Female Hormone Panel - Saliva											
Day of Cycle	Day	2	5	9	11	13	15	17	20	23	26	29
Estradiol	pg/ml	3	3	5	7	12	8	4	8	7	5	3
Progesterone	pg/ml	18	16	13	21	24	67	182	221	155	63	20

Cycle Information	Start 06/14/2015		Ranges	Phase	Estradiol	Progesterone
	End 07/11/2015			Follicular	2 - 10 pg/ml	20 - 100 pg/ml
	Length 27			Preovulatory	7 - 25 pg/ml	
				Luteal	3 - 16 pg/ml	65 - 500 pg/ml

Test	Description		Result		Ref Values
DHEA	Dehydroepiandrosterone Free [DHEA + DHEA-S]	Pooled Value	6	Normal	Adults (M/F): 3-10 ng/ml
TTF	Free Testosterone	Cycle Average	37	Normal	Borderline: 6-9 pg/ml Normal: 10-38 pg/ml

—Image courtesy of Diagnos-Techs, Inc.

Excessive estrogen in the body can cause similar symptoms even when progesterone levels are normal. This is called *estrogen dominance* and should be ruled out when taking blood or saliva samples.

Natural Hormone Therapy

Natural hormone therapy (HT) uses progesterone derived from fermented wild yam. These hormones are bioidentical, meaning that chemically they are exactly the same as the hormones produced by a woman's body. There are many forms of administration available, including sublingual drops, pellets or troches, topical creams, gels, patches, or oral capsules. I have found the sublingual forms to act the quickest. The dosage is easy to control and generally provides symptom relief within 24–48 hours. They wash out of the body quickly, allowing for simple dose changes.

If the woman is not menstruating, progesterone is used daily until her menses returns. This dosing is also appropriate if she has severe symptoms of PMS that persist through day 1 of the menstrual cycle beginning. Women with estrogen dominance may often need to take the progesterone all month long until their bodies are properly supported. It's safe to take progesterone throughout the cycle. Be aware that some women will not begin menstruating until the progesterone is stopped. I advise women to watch for days 28 through 30, and if the menses does not begin, I recommend stopping the progesterone supplementation for a couple of days to see if the flow begins. If a woman has a strong return of symptoms, it's acceptable to resume the progesterone at any time, even while menstruating. When first beginning HT, it's important to keep track of the menstrual cycle.

In menstruating women, the decision of when to begin supplementation with progesterone is based upon symptoms. Most often, a woman will use the progesterone starting on days 12 through 18, until she begins bleeding. Discontinuing the use of progesterone from day 1 (first day of bleeding) till day 12 (ovulation) follows the body's natural rhythm. (see chart above)

As previously stated, if her symptoms begin early in the cycle or do not end with the beginning of menses, she may use the progesterone daily. It's important to follow the advice of a trained physician and monitor blood levels after beginning therapy.

Some women take a smaller dose of progesterone on days 5 through 12 and then increase throughout the month as their period approaches. This cycling mimics the natural rhythm of progesterone in a menstruating woman.

Benefits of Natural Progesterone Therapy

The benefits of natural progesterone therapy include the stabilization of mood, decreased PMS symptoms, and protection from endometrial and breast cancer. Do not use synthetic progestin found in the birth control pills, *Provera,* or *PremPro.* These can cause depression, cancer, and heart disease.

Progesterone also reduces estrogen dominance and decreases anxiety. It's very helpful for treating sleep disorders, night sweats, excessive crying and sadness, delay of menstruation beginning postpartum, or periods that are irregular—either coming too frequently or not at all. It also helps with menstrual cramping and breast discomfort.

Too much progesterone can cause nipple tenderness, and in women who are blood type A, it may cause bloating. Anytime HT is given to a woman, close monitoring of her symptoms and blood levels is important until she has stabilized. It is also important that she is seen by her practitioner weekly until the mood has stabilized. This is especially important if she is having violent thoughts.

Herbal and Homeopathic Remedies

Herbal therapies may be substituted for natural, bioidentical hormones. *Vitex agnus-castus* (Vitex) or chaste tree berry is an excellent choice for younger women. Depending on the severity of the postpartum mood disorder, it may be advisable to begin with HT, and once the symptoms have stabilized, a change to Vitex can be made safely.

Vitex is similar to progesterone in its effect but is not the same as giving progesterone. It takes longer (usually four to six weeks) for the postpartum mood disorder to improve. For this reason, if a woman is severely suffering from PPD or PPMD, regardless of her age, it may be better to begin with HT.

Regarding the use of homeopathic medicines, it would be valuable to have a complete homeopathic intake with a skilled practitioner. Although women may have the same diagnosis, they may need different remedies based on their homeopathic constitution.

In Conclusion

Generally, hormonal imbalances are caused by a deficiency in progesterone levels postpartum. This is not the only reason, but it is the most common cause. Other hormonal imbalances play a part depending on the woman's age and medical history. By finding a competent practitioner to work with you, outcomes can be improved.

It's valuable to look at results from blood tests and rule out other causes. Low blood glucose or iron levels can lead to fatigue and irritability. Other hormone levels—such as estrogen and testosterone—are important for women over thirty-five. When there is severe fatigue or anxiety, testing for the Epstein-Barr virus—as well as DHEA and cortisol levels—may rule out more causes for the symptoms. The thyroid may also be affected postpartum, and thyroid testing will be important in some cases. If the symptoms warrant it, testing for the possibility of Hashimoto's disease or another autoimmune disorder is vital. If the birth experience was very stressful or the home situation is difficult, the adrenals may be taxed by pregnancy. It is important to also conduct adrenal function testing if the new mother isn't feeling better after two weeks of beginning treatment.

Chapter 2

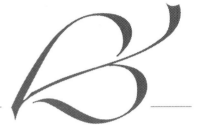

Nutritional Program

Let food be thy Medicine and let Medicine be thy food.
—Hippocrates

The goal of a healthy nutritional program is to insure proper nourishment, keep blood sugar levels stable, and improve digestive function. Organic foods are always preferred over those commercially grown. Incorporating the blood type diet by Dr. Peter D'Adamo will improve results, as will the avoidance of all processed foods and any know allergens.

The Plan

The use of whole foods, which are minimally processed and do not contain preservatives or chemicals, is critical. In all cases, organic is preferred over nonorganic. This will avoid the use of genetically modified (GMO) foods.

Meat: Consuming animal flesh may be helpful for some women to restore health, but is not a necessity. Select free-range, grass-fed, organic, or non-farmed animal products preferably not cured nor smoked.

Fresh vegetables and fruits: When possible, choose frozen over canned.

Whole grains and cereals: The label must say *whole grains*. Avoid processed and refined grains. For example, choose brown rice over white rice. Making half brown and half white rice makes it easier to start eating healthier grains. Whole grain pastas, breads, and cereals are widely available at health food stores.

Organic dairy products: Consume organic whole milk, yogurt, and natural cheeses (avoid low-fat and nonfat). Yogurt naturally sweetened with fresh fruit or honey and vanilla—no sugar or artificial sweeteners. Try goat cheeses and goat yogurts for variety as well as soy, almond, or rice milk. When using dairy, it's important to purchase organic products because of the hormones used in producing nonorganic milk.

Nuts and nut butters: Consume raw nuts, not honey-roasted or sugar-coated. Nuts should be soaked overnight, rinsed, and dried in an oven or dehydrator. This will release enzymes which help with digestion of nuts.

Beans and legumes: For all types of beans and legumes, soak overnight and then rinse in fresh water before cooking to reduce gas or bloating.

Pure water: Drink half your body weight in ounces every day. If you weigh 130 pounds, drink sixty-five ounces of pure water daily. If you are nursing, you will need to drink water more often and in greater quantity.

Herbal teas and sparkling water: These may help you increase your water intake and may be counted as water if only sweetened naturally with honey or stevia.

Getting Started

Begin by eliminating white flours (bread, crackers, and pasta), white rice, and white sugar. The standard American diet (SAD) includes excessive amounts of processed foods made from refined wheat and sugar. The revised *food plate* promoted by the USDA now encourages adding whole grains in addition to processed and refined carbohydrates. By reading the labels on everything you buy, you can eventually learn what to purchase and what to avoid. Look for the words *whole grains, organic,* and *non-GMO certified* when shopping.

What to Avoid

- alcohol, caffeine, nicotine, any street drugs, colas/sodas, coffee, "diet" pills or teas
- white flour, white sugar, white rice, artificial sweeteners, fast food, junk food, chips, cookies, and candies
- hydrogenated oils and preservatives
- GMO, nonorganic, or foods that have been shipped long distances which are often sprayed with chemicals

How to Plan Meals

Eating four to six mini-meals a day reduces the time needed to prepare food. This also keeps the appetite and blood sugar more stable. Many women do not have the patience to eat or cook formal meals. Eating mini-meals allows for meals that can be quickly prepared and eaten upon arising and every few hours through the day.

It's important to incorporate some protein in each snack. Simple examples are:

- rice cake, celery stick, or apple with some nut butter or cheese, tuna, or egg salad on it;
- yogurt or a glass of milk with whole grain granola and fruit. Dairy is a good source of protein if a food allergy doesn't complicate digestion; and
- smoothies made with frozen fruit, coconut water, and protein powder are quick, easy, and nutritious. Check your blood type recommendations or food allergy restrictions before choosing a protein powder. Eggs, whey, and soy

are common allergens. If those are problematic, look for protein powders made from sprouted brown rice, hemp, or pea.

A fresh supply of hard boiled eggs, cooked chicken, organic luncheon meats (turkey, beef, or chicken), canned tuna, nut butters, brown rice cakes and crackers, celery and baby carrots, apples, pears and other fruits, raw nuts, sliced soy cheese, yogurt, and healthy granola bars may be kept on hand. Mix and match all these items for quick and easy snacks.

A carafe of herbal tea may be prepared nightly by soaking four tea bags in a quart of water and refrigerating. Keep sparkling mineral water, purified drinking water, and pure juices in stock.

Not all meals must be of the *mini* variety. For some women, making one meal a day may rarely be possible. However, when time and mood allow, the preparing of a good dinner of protein, salad, and steamed vegetables, with fruit for dessert—or a big breakfast omelet stuffed with meat, sautéed vegetables, and cheese with salsa on top and a whole grain bagel—can be therapeutic. Otherwise, the small snacks will be just fine and adequate for good health.

Eating out requires some planning. Order the protein grilled, baked, or blackened, with a side of steamed vegetables. Hold the starch unless quinoa, brown rice, or sweet potato is available, and of course refuse the bread basket; it is doubtful these items will be whole grain. Another option is to order a salad with protein and the dressing on the side; dipping the fork in the dressing instead of pouring it over the salad will reduce intake of dressings that may contain hydrogenated oils, MSG, sugar, or preservatives. Ordering sparkling water with some cranberry juice or a non-alcoholic beer and skipping the dessert or having fresh fruit is recommended.

Once or twice a week, having something enjoyable that is off the diet will help you stick to the plan better by not having to be perfect. Long-term health and happiness may be better served by taking a break for a day. If a small indulgence triggers binge eating or food cravings, it's best to skip this suggestion.

Remember that what a person does 90 percent of the time is what counts! Three meals a day add up to twenty-one meals per week. Ninety percent adherence to the plan allows for two meals per week off the diet.

Perfection is an illusion and a dangerous one at that. Strive to do well and feel well, not to be perfect.

Why does this diet work?

1. *It stabilizes blood glucose (sugar) levels.* Eating mini-meals prevents the ups and downs of hypoglycemia (low blood sugar). It will keep the metabolism going and reduce feelings of hunger. Eating every few hours rather than waiting to be hungry is the key.

Avoiding refined carbohydrates and sugar will also stabilize the blood glucose levels. Eating sugar gives an initial *boost* that is followed by a *crash* as insulin levels increase. Over time, this can cause insulin resistance and prediabetic conditions.

Repairing the metabolic damage from unstable blood sugar and hypoglycemia, will stabilize mood and improve energy. Over time, it will no longer be necessary to eat so often. As mood stabilizes and energy improves, eating as often may not be as important.

2. *Fueling the metabolism contributes to weight loss.* It's a proven fact that by starving the body, it will hold onto weight. However, by keeping the metabolic fire burning, you will actually lose weight. Most women want to lose weight after giving birth. This is motivation for sticking with the nutrition plan.

3. *Hydration is important for good health.* Drinking two to three liters of water and herbal teas every day will keep the milk supply flowing and prevent dehydration. Dips in blood sugar and dehydration both contribute to depression!

4. *Fats can be healthy.* The increased consumption of healthy fats called *essential fatty acids* is important to good health; the body needs them. Adding one tablespoon of flax oil to a smoothie or pouring it on a salad or steamed veggies just before serving will be beneficial. Flax oil should not be heated. Olive oil is best for cooking and can also be used in salad dressing.

5. *It eliminates pesticides, hormones, preservatives, and other harmful chemicals from the diet.* Removing these toxins will not only restore health, but also it will bring it to a new level. Eating food in its more natural form is the goal and is an easy way to avoid refined and processed foods. This is a lifestyle change to work toward; it's not a temporary fix. Eating more healthfully impacts the health of the entire family and the planet.

Chapter Three

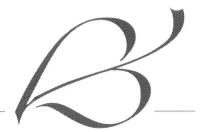

Supplements

I believe that you can, by taking some simple and inexpensive measures, lead a longer life and extend your years of well- being. My most important recommendation is that you take vitamins every day in optimum amounts to supplement the vitamins that you receive in your food.

—Linus Pauling

A high-quality prenatal vitamin is recommended while pregnant and nursing. Many different types exist, and it is advantageous to take one made by a reputable company. Women will often get belching, gas, bloating or constipation from the use of standard prescribed prenatal vitamins. If this happens, it's a sign that a better quality alternative is in order.

Once the baby is weaned, switching to a vitamin specifically for nutritional needs—and based on blood type, preferences, and lifestyle—promotes long-term health. Other supplements may be incorporated depending on particular needs.

Probiotics are generally recommended for healthy gut flora. Often with pregnancy, there is a change in the body's floral balance that may cause problems with bowel function and food cravings. A high-quality probiotic can reestablish healthy colon flora and allow for better assimilation of nutrients as well as improved vitality and wellness.

Omega-3 fatty acids from flax or fish oils can help make the cells of the body healthier. Incorporating essential fatty acids into the diet can also improve the appearance of hair, skin, and nails. They also help with hormonal balance, mood, and memory.

Herbal combinations for sleep, energy, or mood support may be helpful for short-term use postpartum. If you find you need them every day for over a week, take a deeper look at the underlying causes of the symptoms.

The following herbs should be avoided while nursing:

- aloe vera
- basil

- bugleweed
- cascara sagrada
- coltsfoot
- comfrey
- elecampane
- ephedra
- parsley (can dry up milk)
- sage (can dry up milk)
- wormwood

Also avoid any herbs that may be too strong for the baby's digestion, including:

- black pepper
- chili pepper
- garlic
- onions
- oregano
- peppermint

Targeted Amino Acid Therapies (TAAT)

Amino acids are the building blocks of protein. They aren't medications; they naturally occur in foods high in protein.

Neurotransmitters are chemicals the brain makes that affect mood, emotions, and thought processes (cognition). Serotonin is the most well-known of these, as it is affected by medications called *selective serotonin re-uptake inhibitors* or SSRIs; these include Prozac, Zoloft, Paxil, Celexa, and others. Balancing neurotransmitter levels in the brain can affect mental health and cognition.

A simple urine test may be conducted to evaluate neurotransmitter levels. When brain chemistry has been disrupted, this is an important piece of the puzzle. For women who wish to discontinue pharmaceutical medications, this test must be done before changing the medications. Retesting is performed periodically while tapering off the medication, only under a doctor's supervision.

Each course of treatment is completely individualized for the person. Some women respond very quickly and can discontinue the TAAT within a short period of time (less than six months). Others require more extensive testing and treatment, especially if they have a history of depression and use of medications for mood disorders. Not all women go off their medications, and many find that the TAAT will improve the effectiveness of their medications. Prior to reducing any prescription medications, it's necessary to discuss with a trained physician how to taper off the drugs. The tapering should not begin until there is some improvement in symptoms, unless the medications are causing harm.

The treatment protocols allow for symptom relief initially, followed by a stabilizing phase, and then finally a support phase. Each person is an individual and must be treated as such. Some women may eventually wean off the TAAT completely or need to stay on a low dose of nutritional supplements long-term. In neurotransmitter balancing the treatments are always unique and specific to the individual.

Neurotransmitters:

Epinephrine (known as adrenaline) is a neurotransmitter and hormone essential to the body's metabolism. It's important in providing energy, motivation, and mental focus.

GABA is the major inhibitory neurotransmitter in the brain, and an imbalance is associated with increased anxiety and sleep-related problems. GABA provides feelings of calm and relaxation.

Glutamate is the major excitatory neurotransmitter of the brain and at very high concentrations can be excitotoxic, meaning it can damage the brain. It's needed for learning and memory.

Norepinephrine is important for focus and attention. High levels contribute to anxiety and depression. It can be low due to hormonal imbalances and is important for emotional stability.

Serotonin is synthesized by enzymes that act on tryptophan and/ or 5-HTP. Serotonin has been extensively studied as a therapeutic target for depression, compulsive disorders, anxiety, insomnia, and migraines.

Dopamine, a precursor to norepinephrine and epinephrine, plays a significant role in cognitive function and emotion. It provides feelings of pleasure and satisfaction and is also important for muscle function, muscle control, and digestion.

Taurine promotes calmness and is important for proper heart function and healthy sleep.

Glycine, similar to GABA, is necessary for calming and relaxing the body. Relaxing is an important part of healthy sleep.

Histamine controls the sleep-wake cycle, energy, and motivation.

PEA is important in focus and concentration.

Amino Acids:

Glutamine is the most prevalent amino acid in the body. The precursor to glutamate and GABA, glutamine is also important in pH balance, immune function, mental acuity, and carbohydrate cravings.

Taurine is an inhibitory amino acid, counteracting the effects of excitatory transmitters. It decreases stress and anxiety and enhances the effects of GABA.

5-HTP is the amino acid intermediary of tryptophan in the synthesis of serotonin. 5-HTP readily crosses the blood brain barrier increasing serotonin levels in the brain.

Theanine modulates the excretion of serotonin and catecholamines. It is neuroprotective and produces a calming effect to prevent overstimulation. It's commonly used for relaxation, stress reduction, improving learning, mental acuity, and concentration.

GABA is both a neurotransmitter and amino acid. GABA is the major inhibitory neurotransmitter in the brain and is associated with increased anxiety and sleep-related problems. We can consider GABA as trying to put on the brakes when there is an imbalance causing anxiety.

Chapter Four

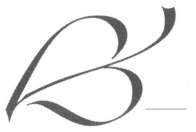

Lifestyle & Exercise

Lack of activity destroys the good condition of every human being, while movement and methodical physical exercise save it and preserve it.

—Plato

1. Cardiovascular Exercise

The cardiovascular system can be improved by raising the target heart rate to 70–80 percent (see the following chart) and maintaining it for at least twenty minutes. Good cardiovascular activities include walking, biking, jogging, treadmills, stationary bikes, elliptical machines, swimming, kayaking, tennis, aerobics, or other sports that will consistently keep the heart rate in the desired zone. Also, staying in the 70–80 percent range during exercise helps burn fat and spare muscle.

You can take your pulse at either your neck (carotid artery) or wrist (radial artery) using your fingers, not your thumb. Counting the number of beats in a ten-second interval every ten minutes during exercise is best.

Finding your target heart rate is accomplished by taking your pulse for ten seconds, finding your age in the left-hand column, and then following across the row to find the ten-second pulse count for 70–80 percent. Keep the target heart rate in the 70–80 percent range during cardiovascular exercise, either increasing or decreasing intensity as needed.

Target Heart Rate Chart

T.H.R.	60%	70%	80%	90%
AGE				
20–24	20	22	24	26
25–29	19	21	23	26
30–34	19	21	23	26
35–39	18	20	21	24
40–44	18	20	21	24
45–49	17	19	20	23

2. Weight, Resistance, and Strength Training

This includes lifting weights, using hydraulic machines, and taking exercise classes designed to increase muscle mass. Weight and strength training will increase lean body mass and raise metabolism. This allows the body to burn more calories without exercising for long periods of time. Muscle is more metabolically active and denser than fat. Although your weight may remain stable, your dress size may decrease.

It's important for women to perform weight-bearing exercise for their bone health. Walking is considered to be a weight-bearing exercise, because it is moving the weight of the body. Weight training can be performed to tone the muscles without creating bulk by increasing repetitions, not weight. Using lower weights will increase strength and make the body appear slimmer, because muscle weighs more than fat but is more compact.

3. Waist-to-Hip Ratio

A simple method for looking at appropriate weight for the frame is the *waist-to-hip ratio*.

Measure the circumference of your waist two inches above and two inches below the belly button; then average these by adding the two amounts and dividing by two. This will give the true waist measurement. Measure the circumference of the hips above the buttocks and at the top of the hip bone (the iliac crest). Then average by adding the two amounts and dividing by two. Divide the average waist circumference by the hip measurement to find the waist-to-hip ratio.

The waist-to-hip ratio should be less than 0.8 for women. A number above 1.0 will cause an increased risk for *metabolic syndrome*, cardiovascular disease, diabetes, and cancer. It's important in looking at overall health and wellness to avoid the risk factors for these diseases and instead bring overall health to a higher level.

4. Lowering Body Mass Index (BMI)

Reducing BMI reduces the risk for many diseases and increases longevity. BMI is computed by dividing weight in kilograms by height in meters squared. (See BMI chart.)

A BMI of 19–24 is desirable, with a waist of less than or equal to 35 inches for women. A BMI of 25–29 is overweight, over 30 is obese, and over 40 is extremely obese. As the waist size exceeds 35 inches in women, the risk for disease is increased.

The table below is used by finding the height in inches on the left column. Move across the row to the weight in pounds. The number at the top of the column is the BMI.

Body Mass Index Chart

BMI	19	20	21	22	23	24	25	30	40
Height inches	Weight in lbs.								
58	91	96	100	105	110	115	119	143	191
59	94	99	104	109	114	119	124	148	198
60	97	102	107	112	118	123	128	153	204
61	100	106	111	116	122	127	132	158	211
62	104	109	115	120	126	131	136	164	218

63	107	113	118	124	130	135	141	169	225
64	110	116	122	128	134	140	145	174	232
65	114	120	126	132	138	144	150	180	240
66	118	124	130	136	142	148	155	186	247
67	121	127	134	140	146	153	159	191	255
68	125	131	138	144	151	158	164	197	262
69	128	135	142	149	155	162	169	203	270
70	132	139	146	153	160	167	174	207	278

5. Stretching

It's necessary to stretch all the major muscle groups, before and after exercising. This can be done by following a simple stretching routine such as the Myrtl Routine. Attending yoga or pilates classes increases muscle mass and provides stretching during the exercise. Comprehensive programs have been created that combine a cardiovascular workout with resistance training in thirty minutes. Finding a convenient, fun, and effective exercise program is an important part of good health and happiness.

In Conclusion:

A good exercise program for health includes:

- exercising three to five times weekly for 20–30 minutes a day;
- raising the target heart rate to 70–80 percent and maintaining it during cardiovascular exercise;
- maintaining a BMI between 19–24; and
- keeping the waist-to-hip ratio under 0.8 for women.

Consistent exercise makes a person feel better in many ways. It releases stress stored in the body by burning up excess adrenaline, releasing endorphins, increasing energy, improving mood, improving the immune system, and enjoying an improved appearance.

Feeling tired after exercise may indicate adrenal imbalance.

Stress-Reducing Strategies

Stress has a strong impact on mood and the immune system. Changing the *response* to stress will improve overall health. It is valuable to remove unnecessary stressors from day-to-day life. Stress is a normal part of life and some of it is healthy. Exercise is an example of a healthy stressor to the body that helps it become stronger. Deadlines for projects can also be positive stress if they push the completion of important work. How a person handles the stress of life is the key.

Implementing some of the following strategies will improve responses to stress and therefore improve health. Some stress-reducing strategies are as follows: meditation (with or without mantra), prayer, yoga, tai chi, qigong, watching a movie, taking a vacation and relaxing, having fun, reading a good book, hanging out with friends, massage, facials, pedicures, manicures, shopping, going out for dinner without children, horseback riding, tennis, surfing, swimming, other sports you enjoy, taking classes, sewing, painting, music, singing, going to museums, and so forth.

The use of aromatic oils can be very soothing to the emotions and body. Inhaling the aromas directly affects the hypothalamus, the part of the brain that controls many endocrine functions in the body.

Lavender:

- calming, relaxing, and balancing
- improve mental accuracy and concentration
- applied topically, may improve hair growth

Frankincense

- diffuse to uplift mood and combat stress
- apply to scars to heal and reduce appearances
- apply to skin to soothe dryness, irritations, and acne

Joy Blend (from www.Young Living.com # 2484020)

- uplift mood and ease anxiety
- overcome deep seated grief
- promote feelings of self-love and confidence

It's important for a woman with postpartum mood disorder to begin connecting with what she enjoyed before the postpartum difficulties began. The more positive action is taken, the more undesirable feelings will be replaced by positive ones. Women often don't realize they have completely stopped doing things they once enjoyed. Starting to add back what PPMD has taken away will need to be a conscious effort at first. Over time, creating a life that is enjoyable and restoring a strong mind and body will bring about the desired health and wellness every new mother deserves.

Chapter Five

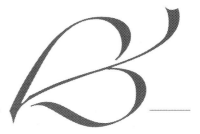

Emotional Support

Our deepest fear is not that we are inadequate, our
deepest fear is that we are powerful beyond measure.
It is our light, not our darkness, that most frightens us.
—Marianne Williamson
(from Nelson Mandela's inaugural speech)

In a traditional society, a woman would have her mother, grandmother, aunts, sisters, cousins, and friends to help her during postpartum. For most women in modern western society, unfortunately, this is not reality. Whether the distance is physical or emotional, not all women have the support of their families. We can create this support network with other women, however.

Many mom's groups have been created to support new mothers. Local government services, schools, and churches are good sources for referrals. For some women, it may be too overwhelming initially to attend these groups. Everyone else may look so happy, and this may create a deeper feeling of aloneness. Self-judgment by comparing a person's inner reality to the outer reflection of others should be avoided. Many women with PPD look like they are doing quite fine to the outside world. It's important to listen to and honor feelings when choosing a group in order to find the right situation. Some groups are designed specifically for women with PPD and have on-line chat rooms as well. It's true that *it takes a village to raise a child.*

A one-on-one relationship with a therapist or counselor may be of great benefit. An understanding person is important to prevent any further shaming or isolation. It's sad to hear some of the comments women are told about their feelings. Find a therapist who is educated.

Feelings are important to show us where a person is off track. When feelings are negative, looking for the causes of discomfort can help find the cause of the pain. Feelings can reveal how certain foods are causing reactions, bringing further knowledge of which foods are beneficial and which should be avoided.

Feelings can help expose who is safe to be around and with whom to share feelings. Following our inner guidance is important for our health and the health of our family. Ignoring, avoiding, or pushing through feelings may create a missed opportunity for healing and growth. Honoring feelings and taking the time to tune in allows for recognition of the next steps to create the lives we crave.

Each person has the answers to all their questions within. Doctors, therapists, clergy, and others are here to help uncover those answers. By supporting and listening to feelings and emotions, these professionals can help.

Physically abusive situations create stress, and action may need to be taken. Some employers may become abusive after a woman has been gone for maternity leave. She may be perceived as having returned in a less productive state. Human resources departments are there to help. Some men may become abusive after the birth of a child. Safety from physical harm for the new mother and child is paramount. If the abuse is verbal, professional help in the form of a counselor, therapist, or psychiatrist may be needed. Words hurt, too, and they can cause harm to the woman and her child. Free help lines are available for women who are being abused.

Sometimes friends and family can be inconsiderate. Many people will want the mother to snap out of it and be grateful for her blessings. Some may want to offer suggestions that may be unhelpful.

One technique is to ask a person to allow the woman to speak about her feelings without any feedback that requires action or is negative. Sometimes all a woman really needs is to be heard.

Chapter Six

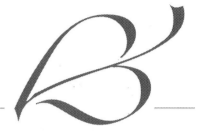

Preventing Postpartum Mood Disorders

An ounce of prevention is worth a pound of cure.
—Benjamin Franklin

The use of naturopathic medicine prior to a woman's pregnancy can contribute to an easier transition and smoother postpartum. Addressing these four main areas prior to conception will lead to a healthier pregnancy and postpartum:

- hormonal balance
- nutrition
- lifestyle
- emotional support

Problems such as infertility, PMS, mood imbalances, weight issues, and other endocrine problems should be addressed before conception to improve health and make necessary change. Avoiding toxins and cleaning up the individual's environment and diet is the best place to start.

Ideally, the health of the male partner should also be addressed prior to conception. Implementing cleansing protocols one to six months prior to conception can improve the health of the sperm. Though a woman is born with all her eggs, a man is constantly producing new sperm. This gives the couple an excellent opportunity to improve the health of the baby by planning to create healthy sperm, eggs, and a parental relationship.

Also, having an understanding partner will improve the quality of support for the new mother. Studies have shown that the partner's support is important, especially in the practical day-to-day help of postpartum. Laying the foundation for a conscious pregnancy and birth experience is necessary to the final outcome of a happy and healthy family.

Some women may begin to have mood disorders during pregnancy. After the first trimester, consider targeted amino acid therapies (TAAT) to prevent a downward slide toward postpartum mood disorders, particularly if depression, anxiety, or mood disorders are in the medical history. It's important to look at confounding factors such as diet, lifestyle, adrenal function, thyroid levels, or autoimmune disorders, as these may be contributing to the problem. Working consciously toward bringing balance and good health before the birth is critical to postpartum joy.

Breanne's Story

Breanne is a twenty-four-year-old with a history of depression that was successfully treated with Zoloft. She is overweight and was smoking and drinking socially until she learned she was pregnant. She was taken off her medication by her MD because of concerns for the pregnancy. She was prescribed a prenatal vitamin with iron. Her chief complaints are depression and constipation.

Neurotransmitter testing revealed low dopamine and serotonin levels. She began TAAT, switched to a high quality, natural prenatal vitamin, and was given dietary suggestions based on blood type. Her constipation resolved shortly after discontinuing the prescribed prenatal vitamin. Within a few weeks her mood had improved and she did well throughout the remainder of her pregnancy.

Two weeks before her delivery date, she began sublingual progesterone and continued her TAAT. She had a healthy baby and no problems postpartum. She nursed the baby for six weeks and then returned to work full-time. She and the baby continued to do well at one year postpartum.

Herbs to Avoid During Pregnancy

Cleansing herbs:

arnica

barberry

bee balm

black walnut

blessed thistle

catnip

chapparal

chicory

coltsfoot

comfrey

ephedra

fenugreek

gentian horehound

horsetail

ipecac

juniper berries

lobelia

oregon grape root

poke root

rhubarb root

rosemary

uva ursi

yarrow

Laxative herbs:

aloe vera

buckthorn

butternut

cascara sagrada

Herbs that affect hormones:

borage

damiana

dong quai

licorice

sarsparilla

siberian ginseng

vitex (can be used the first trimester)

Herbs that cause contractions or bleeding:

angelica

birthwort (bethwort)

black or blue cohosh (can be used the last two weeks of pregnancy)

cotton root

elecampane

fenugreek

feverfew

goldenseal

horehound

lovage

mistletoe

motherwort

mugwort

During pregnancy—more than at any other time in a woman's life—it's best to err on the side of caution. Consultation with a trained professional is vital.

Chapter Seven

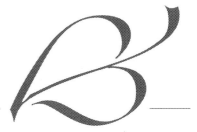

Confounding Factors

*We are what we repeatedly do. Excellence therefore, is
not an act, but a habit.*

—Aristotle

What is the best course of action after:

1. balancing hormone levels
2. changing diet and eating whole foods and mini-meals according to blood type
3. drinking adequate amounts of pure water. Drinking ounces of water equal to half the body weight in pounds. (A 140-pound woman requires seventy ounces of water daily)
4. implementing an exercise and stress reduction program
5. completing proper laboratory testing with a trained professional for analysis of blood, saliva, urine, stool, or hair as needed
6. supplementing proper nutrients to treat any deficiencies
7. getting adequate rest and down time

What if you're still not feeling quite right after doing all of these?

Consider the following possible imbalances:

- food sensitivities
- hypoglycemia/diabetes
- candida/parasites
- anemia (iron or vitamin B12)
- heavy metal toxicity (lead or mercury most commonly)
- endocrine and autoimmune disorders
- low body temperature syndrome

Food Sensitivities:

Foods that cause gastric distress or sensitivity reactions are important to avoid for optimal health. The reactions can be gas and bloating, constipation, diarrhea, skin outbreaks, extreme tiredness, headaches or muscle aches after eating, depression, "crashing" after a meal, or anxiety. For the nursing mother, the baby may show reactions when these foods are eaten. These reactions may include extreme sleepiness, vomiting, gas, colic, diarrhea, skin outbreaks, diaper rash, fussiness, and crying.

The mother's body may stop reacting and no longer show signs of sensitivity because it has habituated to the damaging foods. Over time, humans adjust to foods that are damaging in order to tolerate them with long-term use. Pediatricians routinely tell new mothers with a baby who is vomiting a new formula to continue feeding it and the baby will eventually tolerate it. This is an example of habituation that creates long-term, chronic disease. Avoid foods that cause reactions for mother or baby. A blood test for food allergies or using the naturopathic approach of a challenge/elimination/rotation diet can uncover food sensitivities.

The most reactive foods include:

- wheat
- dairy
- eggs
- sugar
- corn
- caffeine
- soy
- chocolate

Elimination/Challenge/Rotation

How to test for food sensitivities in place of blood testing:

1. Eliminate the suspected food *entirely* from the diet for two to twelve weeks. Find any hidden sources. For example, soy sauce often contains wheat.
2. Reintroduce the food for one day only. Avoid it again for three days.
3. Watch for symptoms over the next three days. If none appear, this food is presumed safe or it was not avoided long enough to bring up the reaction. Begin to rotate this food into the diet, or, if suspicious, resume an additional two weeks of elimination.
4. If symptoms occur such as gas, bloating, constipation, itching, hives, sinusitis, coughing, muscle aches, joint aches, increased cravings, headache, emotional symptoms, or mental confusion—then this food should be avoided for an additional three months before trying to reintroduce.
5. Move on to another challenge, and if no reaction occurs, then reintroduce the food and rotate it into your diet.
6. Rotation means only eating one serving of these foods every three to four days. If symptoms return, avoid the offending food again for two weeks and reintroduce it at longer intervals once a week—or even biweekly or monthly. Eventually, most foods can be rotated into the diet every seventy-two hours.
7. Any food that can't be avoided for two weeks is most likely allergenic.

Dietary Enzymes for a Quick Fix:

If it isn't possible to perform the elimination/challenge/rotation plan, consider this quick fix to the problem. Using the dietary enzymes listed below when eating offending foods can help reduce serious consequences. This is not healing the system, as that requires removing the cause.

1. The dietary enzyme *lactase* may be used if you suspect you are lactose/dairy intolerant. If dairy foods cause gas or bloating, try milk, cheese, and yogurt made from organic sources, goat milk or soy, and take the dietary enzyme lactase. Lactase is available at grocery and health food stores. Use whenever you consume milk products.

2. The dietary enzyme *protease* may be used if meat is difficult to digest. Look for dietary enzymes such as pancreatin or protease.

3. A full spectrum *digestive enzyme* containing lactase, protease, papain, cellulase, and amylase may be used for general difficulties in digestion. I recommend at least one daily with the largest meal. These are available at health food stores.

Substitutions for Common Allergens

If elimination of some foods isn't possible, consider substitutions.

1. *Wheat (including whole wheat)*
Commonly reported effects of wheat allergies are gas, bloating, muscular pain, headaches, and mental confusion.

Switching to sprouted wheat products may reduce symptoms. Spouting grains allows for easier digestion because it breaks down enzyme inhibitors naturally occurring in grains. Other good substitutes are 100 percent rye or rice bread, crackers, and pasta.

Consider eating these products every other day and eating wheat only on special occasions.

2. *Corn*
Corn may be avoided by following the above suggestions. Make sure to read labels, as corn is often a hidden ingredient in many foods.

Watch for high fructose corn syrup in soft drinks and processed foods.

3. *Nuts or beans*
If experiencing gas, make sure to soak beans overnight before rinsing and cooking in fresh water. Nuts may also be soaked overnight, rinsed and then dried in an oven on low heat or a dehydrator. These methods will improve the digestion of beans and nuts. Use an enzyme product such as *Bean-O*, and try different types of nuts and beans.

Increased Intestinal Permeability or *Leaky Gut Syndrome*

Later you may want to test yourself to find if you have any hidden food sensitivities. Some food sensitivities are brought on by increased intestinal permeability. This means that the intestines lose the ability to filter nutrients. This allows food to leak into the blood stream before being properly digested. Substances such as alcohol, sugar, NSAIDs, antibiotics, as well as parasites and other infections can contribute to this condition.

Treatment for weakened digestive tract:

- herbal remedies and nutritional supplements depending on blood type
- L-glutamine: 1,000 mg twice a day
- probiotics (acidophilus/bifidus): twice a day on an empty stomach, preferably taken first thing in the morning and last thing at night.

Use a refrigerated brand of probiotics with live bacteria.

Follow a protocol for at least one month while avoiding the aggravating foods, then retest as above. Some foods may continue to cause problems and need to be avoided beyond this point. You may wish to seek out other forms of alternative treatments to remove food sensitivities such as allergy elimination techniques, homeopathic allergy therapy and acupuncture.

Certain blood types are more sensitive to some foods. Try your blood type diet for a few weeks, and then reintroduce a favorite food you were avoiding. Watch for reactions.

Hypoglycemia & Diabetes:

Hypoglycemia means low blood sugar. It can cause symptoms such as fatigue, restlessness, irritability, dizziness, anxiousness, nervousness, worry, sweating, shaking, trembling, increased pulse rate, racing heart, panicked feeling, shortness of breath, and mental disturbances. It's easier for a nursing woman to go into a hypoglycemic state, since so much of her nutrition is still being given to the baby.

Diabetes can be genetic (juvenile or *type 1*) or caused by lifestyle (adult onset or *type 2*). Many people in the United States are prediabetic or borderline diabetic. A blood glucose tolerance test may show a blood sugar imbalance and can be addressed by diet and exercise. Avoid refined carbohydrates and sugar. Fruit may be eaten in moderation. Eating whole grains, protein, and vegetables in mini-meal format will help stabilize blood sugar levels. Also some women develop gestational diabetes during pregnancy. If this occurs it is beneficial to watch the diet after pregnancy.

You may wonder, *If I have low blood sugar why should I avoid eating sugar?* It has to do with how your body processes the foods you eat. Much of what we eat eventually breaks down into glucose (a sugar) that your body and brain use as fuel. The types of food you eat determine how quickly your body has to convert that food into usable glucose. Whole foods and grains break down much more slowly than processed foods, giving your body the time it needs to digest them properly and make the conversions.

A diet high in sugar will disrupt your body and brain chemistry. When a person eats sugar and refined carbohydrates, it causes blood sugar levels to rise quickly. The body then tries to metabolize this sugar by releasing more insulin. The insulin may lead to a drop in blood sugar from overcompensation. Most people have experienced crashing following a sugar high. This sets a person up for type 2 diabetes (adult onset) due to damage of the pancreas by asking it to work too hard, too often.

Treatment for sugar cravings:

The supplement L-glutamine, an amino acid, can relieve cravings for sugar and carbohydrates.

L-glutamine: 1,000 mg with breakfast and—if cravings are severe—also take a half hour prior to lunch and dinner.

An intense craving may be treated by opening a capsule and dissolving it under your tongue. L-glutamine is slightly sweet in flavor and will cut the craving substantially, hopefully allowing time to make a better choice.

Herbs for Hypoglycemia and Diabetes:

Various herbs may be used to get symptoms and blood sugar levels under control while treating the underlying cause. These vary depending on the individual situation. Herbal combinations can affect blood sugar levels. It's important to be properly monitored by a competent practitioner. Gymnema sylvestre extract for example, has potent anti-diabetic components.

Candida

An overgrowth of yeast in the GI tract can lead to symptoms such as sugar cravings, unexplainable itching, skin rashes, vaginal yeast infections, rectal itching, mental confusion, dizziness, and many other systemic symptoms. Overgrowth can be caused by the use of antibiotics, particularly when probiotics are not administered following a course of antibiotics.

Probiotics help to restore the normal flora in the intestine. When the *good* bacteria are destroyed by the use of antibiotics, opportunistic fungi such as candida can sometimes overpopulate the colon. By using probiotics (the good bacteria such as acidophilus and bifidus), you can repair the damage and bring balance to the colon.

Candida can be ruled out with a blood test or based on symptoms.

Candida Treatment:

1. anti-candida diet: avoid sugar, yeast, mold (cheeses and leftovers), and sweet fruits
2. stinging nettle: take 250 mg with each meal
3. caprylic acid: take 500 mg with each meal
4. garlic capsules: take one with each meal
5. probiotics: take on an empty stomach first thing in the morning and last thing at night
6. IV therapy: intravenous infusions of various substances can eliminate candida in the blood and is recommended in cases of severe imbalance. Please see a doctor who specializes in IV therapy.

Parasites

Rule out with stool sample and treat with herbal tinctures taken two weeks on and one week off throughout the month. Colon hydrotherapy can be helpful in the removal of parasites and nests in the colon. In some cases the use of antifungal or anti-parasitic medications may be required.

Anemia (Iron, Folate, or B12 deficiency)

Rule out with blood test and supplement as needed. Anemia can be caused by the diet or excessive menstruation. It is common in pregnancy due to increased blood volume.

Heavy Metal Toxicity

The major cause of exposure to mercury is silver dental fillings. You may wish to investigate removing these toxic materials from your body. Even a twenty-five-year-old filling can continue to release mercury into the body.

To rule out heavy metal toxicity with urinalysis, a *chelator* can be used as a challenge giving pre- and post- challenge levels. A chelator is a substance that metals bind to in order to be flushed from the body. Chlorella and cilantro are known to be excellent herbal chelators of mercury. Doctors often use DMSA (dimercaptosuccinic acid) which will remove lead, mercury and eighteen other heavy metals from the body. It is not advised to undertake a chelation program without proper medical supervision.

Treatments for heavy metal toxicity may involve using oral or IV chelation therapies. Lead or mercury are the most common toxicities, but toxicity will vary based on individual exposure. Find a doctor who specializes in heavy metal chelation.

If you're undertaking a heavy metal detoxification protocol, it's important that your body eliminate the toxins. If not, you will continue to reabsorb the metals from the bowel. I recommend my patients use some additional methods for detoxification while doing chelation therapies. These methods include colon hydrotherapy, infrared saunas, castor oil packs, and whole-body hydrotherapy.

Endocrine and Autoimmune Disorders:

- Addison's disease
- adrenal fatigue
- hypothyroidism
- hyperthyroidism
- Hashimoto's thyroiditis
- Graves' disease
- Wilson's temperature syndrome
- lupus, Sjögren's syndrome, Rheumatoid arthritis
- Chronic fatigue syndrome/Epstein-Barr virus
- Fibromyalgia

Diagnosing these endocrine disorders requires seeing a doctor or endocrinologist for laboratory testing and evaluation. All of these illnesses are more common in women and may appear postpartum. Natural treatments are available in conjunction with conventional therapies to manage the most damaging symptoms.

Chapter Eight

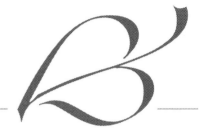

Acute Conditions

First say to yourself what you would be, then do what you would have to do.

—Epictetus

These are some common complaints that may arise following childbirth.

Mastitis

Mastitis is an infection of the breast tissue. It causes pain, swelling, heat, and redness of the breast—and sometimes fever and chills. Lactation mastitis generally occurs within the first three months after giving birth (postpartum) or can develop later during breast-feeding. This condition leads to feeling exhausted and makes it difficult to care for the baby. Often a mother will wean her baby before she intended, due to the pain and exhaustion. It's safe to breastfeed with mastitis. Lactation mastitis tends to affect only one breast.

Signs and symptoms can appear suddenly and include:

- breast tenderness or warmth to the touch;
- generally feeling sick and run down;
- swelling of the breast;
- pain or a burning sensation continuously or only while breast-feeding;
- skin redness, often in a wedge-shaped pattern;
- red streak across the breast; and
- fever of 101°F (38.3°C) or greater.

Conventional treatment usually involves the use of antibiotics and pain relievers. In some cases this may be necessary to avoid an abscess developing in the breast tissue. If the infection stays the same or worsens, a breast exam should be performed by a doctor to rule out an abscess of the breast tissue. This complication can occur when mastitis is improperly treated.

A rare form of breast cancer—inflammatory breast cancer—occurs in 10 percent of breast cancer patients and can also cause redness and swelling that may initially be confused with mastitis. If mastitis isn't better within a week of home care, please seek medical treatment.

- *Natural antibiotic herbs* can help clear up the infection without exacerbating candida, which can contribute to mastitis. Conventional antibiotics can cause candida overgrowth in the bowel.
- *Pain relievers* such as white willow bark and anti-inflammatory herbs such as boswelia, bromelain, curcumin, and quercitin may help reduce pain and swelling.
- *Adjusting the breast-feeding technique can help.* The breasts must be fully emptied during breast-feeding. Often women have issues with the infant latching on correctly. A lactation consultant may review breast-feeding technique for help and ongoing support. Applying warm compresses to the breasts or taking a warm shower before breast-feeding or pumping milk facilitates full emptying. Most hospitals rent more powerful breast pumps than those available in retail stores. Breast-feeding on the unaffected side while pumping the infected breast will bring the best results.
- *Self-care and rest are critical.* Continued breast-feeding, extra rest time, and drinking more fluids will help the body fight the breast infection. With mastitis, it's safe to continue breast-feeding, which adds the benefit of helping clear the infection. Wearing a soft, supportive bra is also helpful. Keep the bra clean and dry.

Hemorrhoids

These are protruding veins near the anus as a result of the pressure from pregnancy and from straining during delivery. Another name for hemorrhoids is *piles*. They can be very itchy and painful and can cause bleeding after pushing during bowel movements. Hemorrhoids can be internal or external, and the symptoms are different depending on the type.

The following classification system is used to categorize the severity of hemorrhoids:

- *first-degree hemorrhoids*: internal hemorrhoids which will bleed but are not prolapsed.
- *second-degree hemorrhoids*: hemorrhoids which will bleed and are prolapsed and will go back to their original state on their own.
- *third-degree hemorrhoids*: hemorrhoids which will bleed and are prolapsed but need to be pushed back with finger.
- *fourth-degree hemorrhoids*: hemorrhoids which will bleed and are prolapsed but cannot be pushed back.

Surgical interventions are generally reserved for fourth-degree hemorrhoids and postpartum due to thinning of the vaginal wall, prolapsed of the bladder (cystocele), injury due to child birth or surgery, and low hormone levels. Below is a comprehensive plan to heal hemorrhoids.

1. *Try to have daily easy bowel movements.* Pushing and straining cause hemorrhoids. Avoid the use of either natural or OTC laxatives if possible. Both can become habit-forming and strain the bowel. Instead, use oxygenated

magnesium to help soften the stool and make evacuation easier. A laxative suppository may be used initially—but only as a short-term remedy. Once the magnesium is working, a small amount of natural lubricant may be used prior to evacuation to make the movement easier and less painful.

2. *Keep the anal area clean.* After evacuation, a sitz bath can be soothing and healing. Put a small amount of warm water in a bathtub and sit for five to ten minutes. Wash the anal area gently and pat dry with a soft towel. The protruding hemorrhoids may be gently pushed back into place, and the area should be cleaned with witch hazel applied to a cotton pad or ball. Other lubricating salves may be applied to soothe and heal.

3. *Strengthen the venous structure.* Collinsonia root is excellent to heal the veins and restore strength to the tissues.

4. *Be aware of dietary changes and food sensitivities.* Though the pressure and pushing of pregnancy may have caused the hemorrhoids, they may persist as a result of reactions to foods. The most common food sensitivities are wheat or gluten, dairy, chocolate, coffee, tomatoes, soy, and corn. Avoiding these foods for one week while using the above bowel hygiene plan should bring rapid results. Once under control, the foods may be reintroduced one at a time every three days. If there is no reaction to the reintroduction, then place that food into a three-day rotation.

Urinary Incontinence

Urinary incontinence is the loss of bladder control. This problem is common during pregnancy because of the weight gain. Incontinence can vary in its symptoms, such as:

- *Stress incontinence*: leaking urine when coughing, sneezing, laughing, exercising, or lifting something heavy.
- *Urge incontinence*: sudden, intense urge to urinate, frequent or involuntary urination, waking to urinate during the night.
- *Overflow incontinence*: dribbling of urine.

Many women are embarrassed and do not seek medical advice; however, it's important to find the cause. Some causes might be:

Reactions to foods and additives. Some foods aggravate the bladder. This cause is ruled out with additional dietary changes. Evaluate the diet for use of alcohol, caffeinated and decaffeinated tea and coffee, and sodas; any of these can trigger incontinence. Remove from the diet artificial sweeteners, corn syrup and other food colorings or preservatives, strong spices, sugar, and citrus fruits.

Urinary tract infections. These can irritate the bladder, causing strong urges to urinate. Symptoms may include a burning sensation and foul-smelling urine. A simple urine test can be performed by your doctor to rule out this condition. The use of cranberry capsules and probiotics can clear up a UTI without further complications of candidiasis from the use of conventional antibiotics. Natural antibiotic herbs such as garlic, ginger, Echinacea and goldenseal can be as effective for clearing infections as conventional antibiotics without the risks.

Constipation. A daily bowel movement is important. Increase the use of probiotics and magnesium to alleviate this issue. If constipation is the cause, urinary frequency and incontinence will resolve themselves.

Prolapse following childbirth. Following a vaginal delivery, the muscles needed for bladder control can become weakened. Kegel exercises can help strengthen the pelvic floor. An internal examination may rule out prolapse of the bladder, uterus, rectum, or small intestine into the vagina. The pelvic floor may also become thinned after pregnancy. The O-Shot is an in-office procedure that uses a small amount of the patient's own blood to rejuvenate the vaginal tissue. It should only be administered by a trained professional. Injecting the platelet-rich plasma (PRP) from the blood into the vaginal canal can help loss of bladder control, sexual dysfunction and pain and restore the integrity to the vaginal wall. See oShot.info

Perimenopause. Many women are having children at an older age, and this can bring on signs of menopause following childbirth. Estrogen and testosterone hormone creams can be applied to the vaginal labia to strengthen the vaginal wall and keep the lining of the bladder healthy and the urethral sphincter strong. Deterioration of vaginal tissues and weak sphincter muscle, can cause incontinence.

Hysterectomy. Surgery can damage pelvic floor muscles, which can lead to incontinence. Kegel exercises can help to strengthen the pelvic floor.

If the cause of incontinence is a thinned pelvic floor as a result of prolapsed organs, decreased hormones or surgery, the O-Shot an in office procedure which uses a small sample of the patient's own blood can help strengthen the pelvic floor and restore the integrity of the tissue. See OShot.info for details on the use of PRP (platelet rich plasma) to restore integrity to the pelvic floor.

Urinary incontinence is a cause of social embarrassment. This unspoken problem further limits enjoyable activities. It contributes to isolation and can increase postpartum mood disorder. It can also lead to increased anxiety in social situations. By finding the cause and receiving proper treatment, this embarrassing hygiene problem can be eliminated.

Chapter Nine

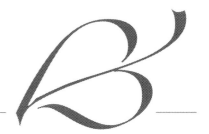

Personal Stories

When you understand that what you're telling is just a story, it isn't happening anymore. When you realize the story you're telling is just words, when you can just crumble up and throw your past in the trashcan, then we'll figure out who you're going to be.

—Chuck Palahniuk

Rachel

Rachel was thirty-six years old when she became pregnant for the first time. She had a history of PMS, depression, and anxiety. She had been treated with extensive therapy and some herbs. She had used birth control pills for over thirteen years and had discontinued all use of contraception for over eight years before becoming pregnant. She had strong beliefs against the use of medications, and though they had been suggested in the past for her mood disorders, she refused anti-depressant medications.

Following the birth of her first child, she began to have violent thoughts and feelings. She was concerned that harm would come to the child and that she might accidentally be the cause of the harm. She had terrible thoughts of the baby being stabbed or dropped from a high place. She was afraid of anything sharp being around the child and asked her husband to hide all the knives and scissors in the house. She clutched the baby tightly if on a balcony or other high place.

Rachel was successfully treated for her postpartum anxiety and obsessive-compulsive thoughts with homeopathy and IV-infused vitamin therapies. She had no problems after about four months postpartum.

At thirty-eight, she became pregnant with her second child. She immediately began to have a hard time, as she was now caring for a toddler, had moved, and did not have the support of a therapist, family, or friends. She developed severe morning sickness, a mitral valve prolapse, a heart murmur, and asthma during the second trimester, which made it difficult for her to function. She again refused medications and instead returned to therapy for her depression and anxiety—which had both worsened.

Following the delivery of her second baby, she felt surreal and detached from it. Although she had felt an immediate bond with the first child, she did not feel that immediate bond with the second. She continued therapy, although it was difficult with a newborn and toddler.

She had very little practical support from her husband and few friends and family. At four months postpartum, she began to suffer from severe depression and anxiety. She had low self-esteem and began to have violent thoughts of suicide and infanticide. The homeopathic medicine made no difference this time.

One evening she was watching a TV program with her husband about Andrea Yates, the woman in Texas who had drowned her five children during a postpartum psychosis. She told her husband about her suicidal and homicidal thoughts, and he encouraged her to speak to her therapist about it and seek other help.

Again, medication was recommended, and though she considered it more seriously now than before, she wanted to nurse her baby and was concerned about potentially unknown side effects. Rachel then sought naturopathic care.

The first step was to look at her hormone levels. At six months postpartum, she was nursing and her menses had not returned. After her first pregnancy menses had resumed at thirteen months postpartum. Saliva tests revealed her progesterone levels to be nearly zero. For some women, this would not be a problem, and lactation would definitely keep progesterone low. For Rachel—with her history of PMS and depression—she needed the hormone.

We began treatment with a natural, sublingual bioidentical hormone preparation made from fermented wild yam. Within five days, she reported a reduction in her emotional instability and an improvement in her self-esteem. She continued this part of the treatment until her menses returned at thirteen months postpartum, the same timing as after her first baby. At that time, we changed the cycling of the hormone to begin on day fifteen through the onset of menses.

Next was the diet. She was eating and drinking very little and had lost much of the fifty pounds she had gained during pregnancy. She had very little appetite and was too anxious to sit down to eat. We created a food plan based on her blood type and encouraged mini-meals that could be eaten quickly and contained high amounts of protein—especially important as she was a blood type O. We also encouraged an increase of her water intake, as dehydration can cause depression.

As for lifestyle, she had begun an exercise program at three months postpartum that she enjoyed. We encouraged a few modifications based on her blood type requirements but generally kept to the plan. We encouraged her to continue therapy and to join a support group of women. This was all helpful to her, and she progressed nicely.

After one year postpartum, Rachel asked that we take her mental health to another level. She still felt depressed and disconnected from the baby. Urinalysis testing of her neurotransmitter levels showed low serotonin, dopamine, and epinephrine. She began a protocol using targeted amino acid therapies (TAAT) and continued to improve.

At sixteen months postpartum she weaned the baby and began to have more problems. Her menses had returned at thirteen months, and she was feeling unwell emotionally and physically despite keeping up with her diet and lifestyle changes. She had created a good support network and was continuing weekly therapy.

Upon further investigation, blood tests revealed a systemic candida infection that had been manifesting throughout the postpartum period as mastitis. She had been treated throughout this time first with three rounds of antibiotics then followed with herbs and diet changes, but she continued to show signs of the overgrowth especially when eating corn products.

Since she was no longer nursing, IV therapy was suggested. She could now approach the problem more aggressively. Each successive treatment yielded improvements in her symptoms. In fact, she had four IV treatments during a six-month period.

Her body temperature had been low for most of her life and was now averaging 96.5°F. She was referred to a doctor for Wilson's temperature syndrome treatment to bring her temperature back to normal. She was on T3 therapy for a full eighteen months before her temperatures reached 98.6°F. This brought about a huge shift in her symptoms. Because much of the body chemistry is due to enzymatic reactions, having a low average temperature is not optimal.

In searching for the cause of the low body temperature syndrome, urinalysis revealed heavy metal toxicity. She did a few months of chelation but was unable to keep up the regime. The heavy metals continue to be a source of her health challenges until she moved to a new location and her exposure decreased. After a few more chelation therapies she cleared the metals and all the symptoms disappeared.

Now at over ten years postpartum, Rachel is doing well. She feels connected to her children and her life in a deep and meaningful way. She has thrived in her career and balances that with family time. She continues the blood type diet and her support group, and she updates her supplements as needed. Rachel is preparing for a smooth transition into menopause and recently added estrogen cream to her regime.

Yvonne

Yvonne is twenty-six years old. At three months postpartum, she was having a rough time emotionally and physically. Extremely depressed with anxiety and paranoia, Yvonne could not care for herself or her baby. She had been completely overwhelmed by a traumatic birth experience.

Though very healthy during the pregnancy, she had a history of depression and emotional abuse. She was married and in a great relationship with a very supportive husband. They ate a healthy, natural diet and lived on an organic farm. She had planned a home birth and had prepared with a *doula* (a woman who supports the mother during labor). She thought it would be easy to have a natural, vaginal delivery.

Instead, her labor would not progress, and she ended up with an emergency Caesarean section. She was very upset about the C-section and felt like a failure. She felt shame around the birth and did not want anyone to know about it. She could not sleep well even when the baby slept. The cries of the baby were excruciating for her. She was suffering from a form of post-traumatic stress disorder (PTSD).

Her MD suggested she stop nursing and begin taking anti-depressant medications. Since she wanted to nurse her baby, she saw a naturopathic doctor but was dissatisfied with that visit. She did not want to change her diet since she thought it was already good, and she was financially unable to pay for any supplements or services.

The following plan was suggested:

1. sublingual progesterone
2. blood-type diet with Candida restrictions
3. neurotransmitter testing

Due to financial concerns, she used a progesterone cream covered by insurance. (Often it will take over two weeks for a woman to begin feeling the effects of a topical cream.)

She did not want to alter her diet. She was smoking marijuana and drinking but didn't think it was a problem. Often women with self medicate with alcohol and marijuana when feeling anxious and depressed. Unfortunately, this self medicating leads to an increase in depression and anxiety. This is due to the rebound reaction of alcohol causing a spike then drop in blood sugar and marijuana causing symptoms of withdrawal. She refused a neurotransmitter test and instead wanted to use amino acids based on her own research. From my experience it is less expensive to take the urine test rather than wasting time and money taking unnecessary supplements.

Her husband called me in complete despair two weeks later, and I made a house call. She was locked in the house and was neglecting the baby and herself, no longer eating or nursing the baby.

She began the sublingual progesterone and eventually discontinued the cream. This led to a great improvement in her despair and paranoia. She was unable to implement the blood-type diet, but she did begin to chart how foods made her feel and noticed she had reactions to the foods that were recommended to avoid for her type.

She took the neurotransmitter test and the results showed that her serotonin, norepinephrine, and epinephrine levels were very low. Her dopamine and GABA were high in response. This biochemical imbalance was causing her to be tired, depressed, anxious, sleepless, and to have uncontrolled thoughts.

We began a targeted amino acid therapy protocol. She followed it for a short time, got relief, and was able to function at a reasonable level. After one year postpartum she was doing very well. She traveled with her husband and child, began to pursue her education, and was quite happy. She then got pregnant for the second time.

I saw her in a social situation and was quite concerned by her outlook on this second pregnancy. She was planning to have a VBAC (vaginal birth after Caesarean) at home and thought this pregnancy would heal the scars of the last one.

I suggested we begin making plans for her future pregnancy and delivery. I agreed that we should be positive and hope for her desired outcome this time. I suggested she schedule a visit with me.

She agreed that she was trying to deny the past and needed more prenatal care. She agreed to see an MD and make plans for a hospital birth with the possibility of a vaginal birth. She was happy just to have the option. We retested her neurotransmitter levels, and I again suggested the blood type diet.

Her tests revealed low serotonin, dopamine, norepinephrine, and epinephrine levels. Her GABA levels were normal. She was not yet beginning to compensate for the imbalances. Her mood was reasonably good, though she was having some anxiety, exhaustion, and frustration. We began her personalized TAAT protocol and sublingual progesterone at very low doses in order to begin supporting her biochemical balance.

We continued to support Yvonne throughout her pregnancy. She retested her neurotransmitter levels and stayed with the suggested TAAT. More dietary and lifestyle changes supported her health. She did have problems with infections caused by flora imbalances, but generally her mood was good.

Her second pregnancy also resulted in a C-section. This time—as a result of all the work she had done in preparation—it didn't feel like a failure. In fact, she reported the experience to be healing, and she did quite well postpartum.

Noel

Noel is twenty-eight years old and spoke with me following a miscarriage that may have also been medically induced. She is married, lives with her in-laws, has a history of depression, and is a survivor of child abuse. She has a thyroid disorder and was being treated by a naturopathic doctor with natural thyroid. She was exhibiting symptoms of PPD at this time. She felt very powerless about her situation and greatly wanted to have a child. She complained of being overweight and tired.

I suggested neurotransmitter testing, and she began the protocol immediately. She was very compliant and stayed with her plan. She made lots of changes in her life and was working on issues from her childhood, especially with her mother who had died. She continued to see me and did quite well, becoming emotionally stronger and happier.

She then became pregnant and was very anxious and afraid of losing the pregnancy again. We talked about this and she read the book *Motherless Mothers* by Hope Edelman. She did quite well after the first trimester and had a healthy pregnancy and delivery.

One week postpartum, Noel returned for an appointment. We had planned for her to return at six weeks postpartum. She was very upset, overwhelmed, crying, and scared. We talked about her symptoms, and she admitted to having thoughts that were very frightening to her. I assured her that other women had these same thoughts and that she would not act on them. I affirmed what a good mother she was and how she loved her child so much that she had come for help immediately.

She felt she hadn't "done it right," because she had accepted pain medication during labor. The medication had caused her to be violently ill with nausea and vomiting, and she regretted the choice. I confirmed that she had done her very best in the moment and that the outcome was in fact perfect—a healthy mom and baby.

We continued her progesterone support and TAAT. I suggested some changes, but immediately following the visit, she felt relieved and confident. I spoke with her by phone twice over the next week. She was doing well and did not feel the need to add the new supplement I had recommended for her anxiety. She continues to do well.

I would like to comment on this point about the irrational thoughts women have postpartum. There seems to be a universal theme of uncontrolled violence. These feelings may spring from a collective unconsciousness. Many women are afraid to be around knives or scissors, as they are afraid they will hurt the baby accidentally. Often there is a fear of high places and that the baby will fall from the balcony, or she will lose control and throw or drop the baby. There may be other violent thoughts of crashing the car, hurting the baby without wanting to, or leaving the baby somewhere by accident. It's important that these women be evaluated and supported nutritionally, emotionally, and biochemically. Following proper evaluation, they can be assured that they are not going to act on these thoughts. As I told Noel, it's a wide spectrum from baby blues to postpartum mood disorder to psychosis. Because she was given the proper support, I feel we have avoided PPD in Noel—and she experienced a normal blue spell that lasted only a few days and resolved with emotional support and continued physical supplementation.

Conclusion

In the practice of naturopathic medicine, searching for the cause of the illness and, if possible, removing the cause, are of utmost importance.

There are times when treating the symptom is necessary in order to give relief from suffering, bring comfort, and stabilize a situation while the underlying cause is addressed. There are times when the cause cannot be removed and time must pass in order for change to occur and healing to begin.

Symptoms are the body's way of trying to get attention. "Look something is wrong here!" it tells us. Sometimes a symptom is an isolated incident, and removing the symptom is enough. However, chronically covering up symptoms not only makes the cause more difficult to find, but also it compounds the problem.

Look at the example of a headache. Aspirin may remove the symptom of the headache, but unless the cause is addressed, repeated use of aspirin can create another illness—an ulcer!

My hope in writing this book is to minimize the suffering of women by encouraging them to seek and get appropriate treatment early in the illness. I hope the stigma of postpartum mood disorders will be lessened by education replacing ignorance, and that ultimately women will be able to find good health throughout their reproductive years and avoid PPMD altogether.

In health,
Dr. Nancy Lins, ND
August 16, 2014
Lahaina, Hawaii

Resources

ALCAT
For food allergy testing
www.ALCAT.com

DiagnosTechs
For hormone testing
www.diagnostechs.com

Doctor's Data
For heavy metal testing
www.doctorsdata.com

Genoma (4 Your Type)
For blood type information
www.4yourtype.com

Genova
For hormone testing
www.gsdl.com

ImmunoLabs
For food allergy testing
www.ImmunoLabs.com

Natural Partners
For quality supplements
www.npscript.com/aliiwellness
access code: drlins

NeuroScience
For neurotransmitter testing
www.neurorelief.com

OShot
For incontinence and sexual dysfunction
www.OShot.info

Post Partum Support International
For information on PPD
www.postpartum.net

Wilson's Temperature Syndrome
For information on low body temperature syndrome
www.WTSmed.com

Young Living Oils
Essential oils and supplements
www.youngliving.com #2484020

Bibliography

Ahlgrimm, Marla, R.Ph., Kells, John M., Rodgerson, Christine Mcgenn. *The HRT Solution*. USA: Penguin Group Inc., 2003.

Briggs, B., Freeman, R., Yaffe, S. *Drugs in Pregnancy and Lactation*. Baltimore, MD: Lippincott Williams and Wilkins, 1998.

Cass, Hyla, MD. *St. John's Wort, Nature's Blues Buster*. Garden City Park, NY: Avery Publishing Group, Inc., 1998.

Dalton, Katharina. *Depression After Childbirth*. Oxford, New York: Oxford University Press, 1989.

D'Adamo, Peter J.D. *Live Right For Your Type*. USA: Penguin Putnam Inc., 2001.

Hudson, T. *Woman's Encyclopedia of Natural Medicine*. Los Angeles: Keats Publishing, 1999.

Larson, Joan Mathews. PhD. *Depression-Free, Naturally*. New York, USA: Ballantine Publishing Group, 1999.

Lucille, Holly, ND, RN. *Creating and Maintaining Balance*. Boulder, CO: IMPAKT Health, 2004.

Oday, P. *Herbs for a Healthy Pregnancy*. Los Angeles, CA: Keat's Publishing, 1999.

PDR for Herbal Medicines. Montvale, NJ: Medical Economics, 1998.

PDR for Nutritional Supplements. Montvale, NJ: Medical Economics, 1998.

Reiss, Uzzi., MD, OB/GYN. *Natural Hormone Balance.* USA: Pocket Books, 2001.

Romm, S. *Natural Health After Birth.* Rochester, VT: Healing Arts Press, 2002.

Wilson, Denis E., MD. *Wilson's Temperature Syndrome.* Lady Lake, Florida: WilsonsTemperatureSyndrome.com, 2005.

References

Ahokas, A., et al. 2001. "Estrogen Deficiency in Severe Post Partum Depression, Successful Treatment with Sublingual Physiologic 17 beta-estradiol." *Journal of Clinical Psychiatry* May, 62 (5):332–336.

American Academy of Pediatrics Committee on Drugs. 2001. "The Transfer of Drugs and other Chemicals into Human Milk." *Pediatrics* 108 (3):775–789.

Bhatia SC, Bhatia SK. 2002. "Diagnosis and treatment of premenstrual dysphoric disorder." *Am Fam Physician* 66(7):1239–48.

Bloch, M., et al. 2000. "Effects of Gonadal Steroids in Women with History of Post PartumDepression." *American Journal of Psychiatry* June; 157 (6):924–930.

Gregoire, A.J., et al. 1996. "Transdermal Estrogen Effective Treatment for Post Natal Depression." *Lancet* April 6: 347 (9006): 918–919.

Harrer G., Sommer H. 1994. "Treatment of mild/moderate depressions with Hypericum." *Phytomed* 1:3–8.

Laakmann G, et al. 1998. "St. John's Wort in mild to moderate depression: the relevance of Hyperforin for the clinical efficacy." *Pharmacopsychiatry* 31(suppl. 1):54–9.

Thys-Jacobs S, Alvir MJ. 1995. "Calcium-regulating hormones across the menstrual cycle: Evidence of a secondary hyperparathyroidism in women with PMS." *J Cline Endocrinol Metab* 80:2227–32.

Index

About the Author

Dr. Nancy Lins is a board-certified naturopathic physician licensed in Hawaii. She received her doctoral training from the Southwest College of Naturopathic Medicine and Health Sciences in Tempe, Arizona. That training included a four-year didactic program and clinical residency. Her studies included the use of various natural modalities—including nutrition, IV vitamin therapies, botanical medicine, homeopathic medicine, natural hormone replacement therapy, acupuncture, structural therapy, and mind/body medicine. Dr. Lins completed her clinical training in Hawaii with Dr. Michael Traub, ND, while he was President of the American Association of Naturopathic Physicians. During that training she focused primarily upon women's health issues pertaining to hormonal imbalances and anti-aging medicine.

Over a two-year period Dr. Lins developed a comprehensive treatment plan for premenstrual syndrome (PMS), Postpartum mood disorder, perimenopause and menopausal symptoms using nutrition, bioidentical hormone replacement, botanical (herbal) medicine, and targeted amino acid and vitamin therapies to heal the body, mind, and spirit.

Dr. Lins began her medical career in Kailua-Kona, Hawaii where she owned and operated a multidisciplinary medical office integrating naturopathic physicians, medical doctors, acupuncture, massage, colon hydrotherapy, and digital infrared imaging for early breast cancer detection.

The mother of two children and married over twenty years, her current practice at Ali'i Wellness is located in Lahaina on Maui. While she is focused on helping women balance their hormones, she also enjoys yoga, nature, and travel.

Visit Dr. Lins' website at www.DrLinsHawaii.com.

Printed in the United States
By Bookmasters